Medical Marijuana –

A Patient Guidebook

Dr. Stephen Blythe

ISBN-13: 978-1511939331

ISBN-10: 1511939338

DEDICATION

This book is dedicated to those whose suffering is met by silence from their providers and from the FDA. It is dedicated also to those who attempt to bring forward a rational discussion of the realities of medical marijuana – happy with the benefits while fully aware of the risks.

Introduction

As a board-certified family physician and nutritionist I have studied plant medicines for the past thirty years. Most of the herbal medicines that patients use have a modest impact for a few very specific conditions. Fresh feverfew will sometimes stop a migraine in its tracks. It may even have a role in prevention of altitude-associated headaches. Echinacea may boost immunity to respiratory viruses. Saw palmetto seems to help about half of my male patients with prostate problems. Yohimbe bark was reputed to help erectile dysfunction – but when there was a prescription product containing this plant medicine, none of those to whom I prescribed it ever requested a refill, so its impact must not have been very significant.

But no plant medicine has the potential helpful impact – sometimes dramatically helpful – across such a range of health problems as does marijuana. I have provided medical marijuana certification for patients in Maine for the past several years, and have seen patients achieve such benefit from this plant that I am now dedicating much of my time to helping qualified patients obtain and use medical marijuana.

Marijuana is not without controversy – the FDA has refused for decades to allow it to be studied as a medicine. It is the fault of the FDA that the current status of marijuana as a medicine is confused and chaotic. The FDA stance on medical marijuana has prevented scientists from doing the kind of research needed – and yet it is the lack of objective research that detractors claim as a reason to shun marijuana as a medicine.

This book is for my patients – and any other patients who would like to understand medical marijuana.

Chapter 1: Plant Medicines

I have to laugh when people tell me that they do not believe in plant medicines – as they sip their coffee (or puff on a cigarette). The World Health Organization estimates that three out of four humans on the planet rely on plant medicines partly or totally. When our newest pharmaceuticals can cost upwards of $800 per month for 30 tablets (Abilify© is a good example) it is easy to imagine that they are beyond the reach of most of the people on earth. The medicinal value of certain plants has been known for eons. Many of our most important medicines today are derived or were originally derived from plants. Examples include the heart medicine digitalis, from the foxglove plant, and colchicine, used for gout, originally derived from the colchicum, a crocus-like flowering plant.

And without quinine, the British Empire would have never amounted to anything. The story of quinine is fascinating. A Jesuit missionary named Agostino Salumbrino working in Lima, Peru learned that the locals would effectively treat a fever by drinking

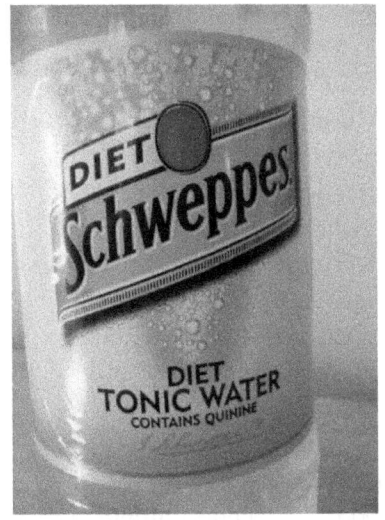

a tonic which they made by soaking the bark of the cinchona tree in water and adding a little sugar to counter the bitterness This seemed to work very well, and in 1631 he sent news of this and samples of cinchona bark back to Rome to see if it would work against the malaria that was plaguing the Mediterranean. It turned out that a compound in this bark (quinine) was very effective in treating and preventing malaria. In 1783 a company named Schweppes created a tonic from this plant and sold it to prevent malaria. This enabled the British to colonize

Medical Marijuana

India and large parts of Africa. Although malaria has become mostly resistant to quinine, this is why Schweppes Tonic Water is today the oldest still-used carbonated beverage!

It was long known that the inner bark of certain plants contains compounds called "salicylates" which lower fevers and help pain. Four hundred years B.C. Hippocrates described using willow bark to treat headache, pain, and fevers. French scientists extracted salicylic acid from the inner bark of the spirea plant – also called meadowsweet - and called this compound "spirin". But this compound was very hard on the stomach, and so chemists with the Bayer Company in Germany attached a chemical group called an "acetyl" group to the spirin, resulting in acetylsalicyclic acid, which they dubbed "a-spirin". To

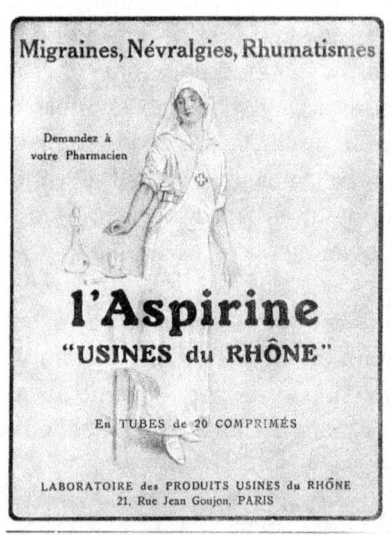

this day it is one of the most widely used medicines on earth.

My first experience with raw plant medicines happened in Peru many years ago. Like many people, whenever I travel to high altitude I get severe headaches. In Peru this is called "soroche". To see the ruins in the Andes you have to travel to the city of Cusco. Cusco sits at the bottom of a valley at 11,300 feet above sea level. Tourists wander the city, gasping for air. The better hotels have oxygen available.

The first day in Cusco I was exploring the ruins just outside of town (Up the mountainside!). An elderly Quechua gentleman asked if I would like him to show me around. He was asking for the equivalent of a dollar, and I said: "Si". As we were walking

2

around, and I was trying to follow his Spanish, I was having a terrible headache. I asked him to slow down, explaining that I had "soroche muy malo". He said: "uno momento" and began looking in the nearby weeds and bushes. He found what he was looking for – "aqui, aqui" he shouted ("here, here"). What he found was a small bush in the mint family. He demonstrated that I was to crush the leaves and inhale the vapor. I did so, and within seconds of breathing in the minty vapor the pain in my head was

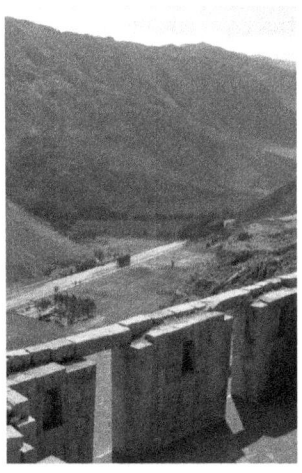

gone! He advised that this effect would only last five or ten minutes, and so I stuffed my pockets with these leaves and could be seen for the next few days wandering the streets of Cusco, my hand to my nose.

At first I had thought he was looking for coca plants. The Quechua of the high Andes have always used coca, which is a safe mild stimulant (until the active ingredient is extracted and concentrated into cocaine), to help them survive the high altitudes. It gives them a little extra energy, and probably helps counter some of the effects of low oxygen levels. Most of the cafes in the Andes sell coca-leaf tea to the tourists, who all think it

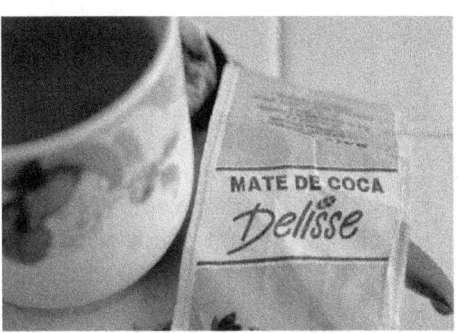

is pretty neat to be drinking legal "mate de coca". However, what most of them don't know is that it is useless – the coca alkaloid compound that is needed is NOT soluble in water! The Quechua will wrap a coca leaf around some crushed limestone or bone meal or ash and place this in their cheek and hold it. The alkalinity of the ash converts the coca alkaloids into a form that can be absorbed into the bloodstream, and they slowly get some benefit from this plant.

Years later I was on a trip to the rainforests of Costa Rica with James Duke, PhD. He is a botanist famous for his research into rainforest medicines – and author of "The Green Pharmacy". I was telling him of my experience with this

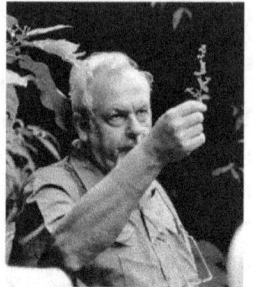

plant, and he said that he had heard of that plant, and that it was indeed in the mint family, and that it was called muño. Like many plant plants with known medicinal properties, it has never been studied. Perhaps it would have great use as a treatment for migraine headaches.

How do plants become medicines?

Tradition: The knowledge of many plant medicines has been handed down from generation to generation. Some of this information has been recorded in ancient written texts, such as in India, China, and Greece. Some has been oral tradition. Such is the example of digitalis. Digitalis is a medicine derived from the foxglove plant – a pretty biannual flower found in many gardens. A British physician first published the use of digitalis to treat "dropsy" – congestive heart failure – in 1785. Although he received acclaim for "discovering" this medicine, he later acknowledged that he was told about it by a village midwife.

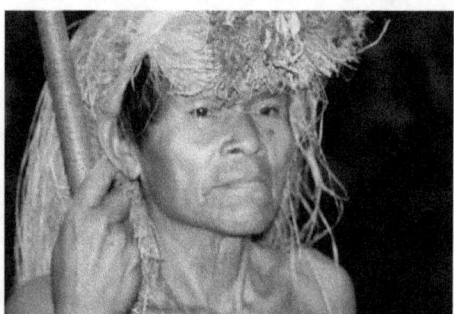

This Yagua hunter in the Amazon uses plants both to ward off mosquitoes and uses a potent mix of plants and frog skin for poisonous darts with which to hunt monkeys and other bushmeat.

Medical Marijuana

When I lived outside of Denver on the "high prairie" of Colorado, I catalogued the plants that grew on our five acres that had been historically used as medicines. Some, such as Echinacea, are still used. Among the wild flowers and "weeds" on our little piece of ground we had over 55 plants that had known medicinal value. Why aren't they still in use? Many reasons – bloodroot, for example, was used to treat parasites – but it caused bad diarrhea. We have better treatments now. Many of the medicinal uses of these plants were shared with the settlers by Native Americans.

"Ethnobotany": While we have learned a lot about traditional plant medicines used by the earliest inhabitants of Europe, the Middle East, and North America, what about other cultures with which we do not have a long history? Many people have traveled to the relatively unexplored regions of the earth for the specific purpose of learning about what local plants are used for what medicinal purpose. This is called "ethnobotany". Dr. Jim Duke, as the director of the USDA's program to search for cancer-treating plants in the rainforest, spent many years traveling through the Amazon and Central America – interviewing shamans and studying the local flora. Some botanists apprenticed themselves to shamans with whom they studied for many years. Vast amounts of information came from these studies.

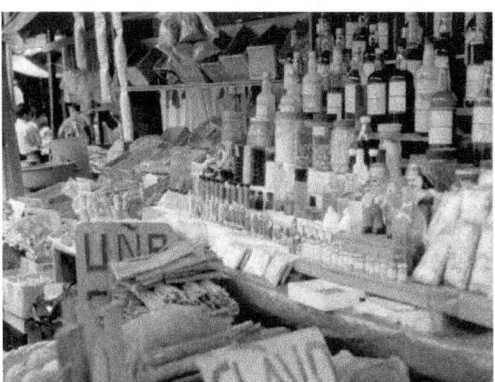

The plant medicine marketplace in Iquitos, Peru, is one of the largest and most fascinating in the world. Bark, roots, leaves, tinctures, and all types of preparations of plant medicines are available.

Medical Marijuana

"Phytomedicinal prospecting": There is actually an organized effort to learn about the biological activity of different plants in several countries. At the Institute for Biodiversity in Costa Rica, for example, they collect plants from all over their country. Extracts of these plants are made and the extracts are tested for antibacterial properties, antiviral properties, anti-cancer properties, anti-parasite properties, and even anti-HIV properties. Any plants showing promise are then studied further.

"Doctrine of Signatures": This is a philosophy through which some people feel we are directed by a higher power to find plants with medicinal values. A leaf that looks like a kidney might be good for kidney problems, for example. Although I think this is somewhat fanciful, there is at least one very good example where it works. The ripe fruit of the saw palmetto plant contains compounds which help treat urinary difficulties in men with enlarged prostate glands. Why were these berries ever tried in the first place? If you find the ripe black berries of the saw palmetto and squeeze them, the juice not only looks like urine, but it smells like urine as well! (Actually it smells like old urine – like you would smell in a New York City subway entrance….).

The Intersection of Plant Medicine and Big Pharma

The story of plant medicines and big pharma can be told by the history of the Mexican Yam (*Diascorea Mexicana*). The Mexican Yam is not a little sweet-potato thing – it is a giant tuber that grows in the jungles of southern Mexico and Central America. I had the opportunity to interview a village midwife in Belize – "Miss Hortense" (she was 84 years old and had been helping pregnant women for 73 years!) and she described how she uses the Mexican Yam for her patients.

It was discovered long ago that this tuber contains the chemical compound diosgenin, a "steroid ring", which could easily be used by pharmaceutical companies as a chemical building block to create all sorts of powerful hormone drugs such as cortisone, estrogen, and testosterone.

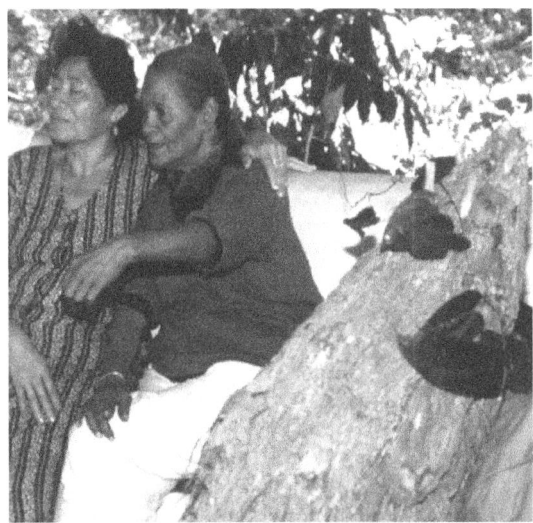

Ms. Hortense with a huge freshly dug tuber of the *Diascorea mexicana*, or "Mexican yam"

Although various products containing Mexican Yam can still be found at health food stores, they probably have little effectiveness without chemical alteration. Mexican farmers were encouraged to grow this plant, and the pharmaceutical industry bought all they could grow. Along came organizers, who suggested that these farmers should start a cooperative – a union – to negotiate better prices for their crops. About that time the pharmaceutical industry finally figured out how to synthesize steroid rings in the factory. So almost overnight the farmers were told they were no longer needed, and almost all steroid compounds are now completely synthesized.

Synthetic drugs can be a huge convenience. Sometimes they can have advantages – as in the case of digitalis. When the leaves of the foxglove plant were first used as medicine, it was quickly realized that the margin between a therapeutic dose and a toxic dose was relatively small – too much and you could die. But with a plant medicine this is a problem. The leaves from one plant could have much different potency than the leaves of another plant

Medical Marijuana

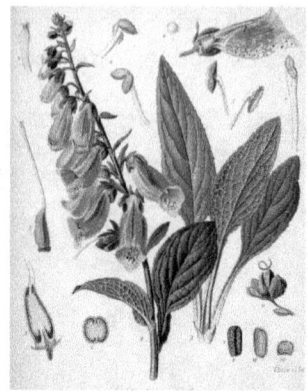

grown in different soil, different light, different moisture, etc. Plants from the sunny side of the hill might be different than plants from the shadier side of the hill. The challenge was how to figure out what the right amount of dried leaf to put in a capsule so that the strength would be consistent and predictable. The answer came with the discovery that pigeons were very sensitive to digitalis leaf – a certain amount was sure to kill a pigeon. So an assay, or test, of the strength of digitalis leaf was developed based on how much it took to kill a pigeon. A large batch of digitalis leaves could be dried, crushed, and blended, and then the strength determined by the pigeon test. This would let the drug-maker know just how much leaf to put in each capsule. It is much easier – and perhaps safer - these days to just synthesize the main active compound, digoxin, and to have the patient take a 0.125mg tablet every day – but we also must check blood levels to make sure the patient is getting the right amount.

But what makes it unlikely that we will see many new drugs derived from plants is the lack of profit. A drug company has to be able to patent a drug in order to charge $10 or more per tablet. A medicine extracted from a plant cannot be patented – and anyone can grow the plant. Medical marijuana is a good example. The FDA continues to insist that there is "no medical use for marijuana" and they classify it as a Schedule I drug – meaning that it has "No medical value or the risk so far outweighs any medical value that it cannot be used". Right alongside crystal meth! However, they allowed Solvay Pharmaceuticals to produce a synthetic THC for treatment of cancer-associated pain, nausea, and weight-loss. This medication, called Marinol, is a Schedule III drug – meaning that it has an "accepted medical use" and has a small to moderate risk of dependence. Marinol, by the way, sells for about $1400 for sixty capsules (enough for a month). Still illegal (at the federal level) to grow your own, though! This should not surprise anyone, since the commissioners of the FDA are generally former pharmaceutical company executives, and big pharma spends lavishly in support of our representatives in Washington, D.C. – the best that money can buy!

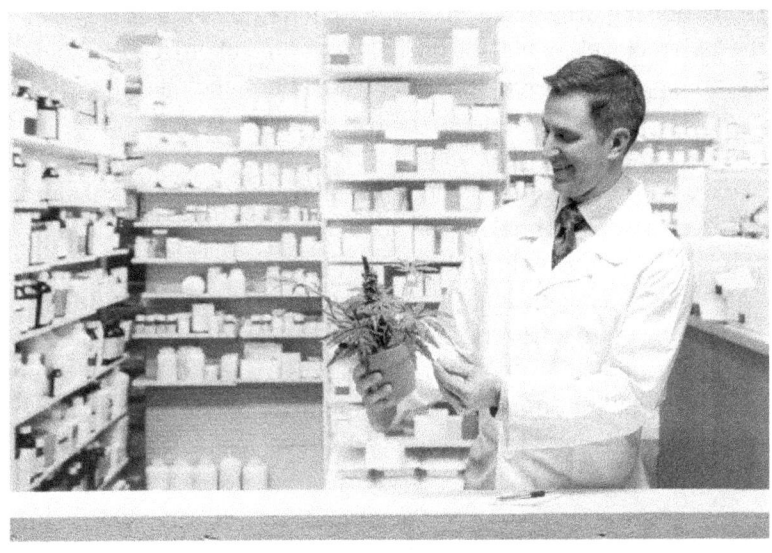

Someday marijuana will be recognized as the medicine that it is!

Chapter 2: Legal Marijuana?

"It's legal – how come I got busted"?

At the time of this writing, almost half the states in the U.S. have made marijuana legal for medical use, and several have made recreational marijuana legal. But marijuana still remains illegal at the federal level. While it is unlikely that the FBI or DEA are going to show up at the door of a marijuana patient and place them under arrest, it could happen. I always remind patients when doing a consultation that they must NOT take their marijuana any place where they would be under the jurisdiction of **federal law enforcement personnel,** or they could face federal prosecution. This would include military bases, national parks, and airports. And while you might simply get a citation and have to pay a fine for lighting up to enjoy the sunrise at Acadia National Park here in Maine, if you had just been to the dispensary and purchased your state-allowed maximum of two and one-half ounces of marijuana, you could be in for a felony arrest and be facing very hard time.

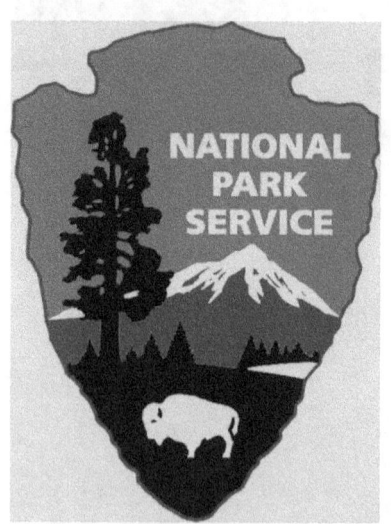

An AP story in January of 2015 states that the U.S. Attorney's office in Wyoming prosecuted 21 people for possession of marijuana in Yellowstone National Park in 2010 – and in 2013 that number was 52, and by December of 2014 the number had risen to 80. Nationwide, thousands of people are arrested yearly for possession of marijuana on federal lands.

Medical Marijuana

In Wyoming these arrests meant a $1,000 fine and a lifelong record for a misdemeanor arrest.

In more pot-friendly California, the fine may be only $350 (sometimes less for those with a medical card), but the potential penalties for a federal-level violation are six months in prison and a $5,000 fine – and that is for a SMALL amount of marijuana!

Since federal law trumps state law, possession of a state-issued medical marijuana certificate or card is generally irrelevant. A federal judge may even deny possession of such a card as a defense for someone wishing to challenge their arrest. No such challenge has happened in my state of Maine that I am aware of - I would find this to be an interesting legal case to watch unfold: but I would not want to be the defendant! Even if you won, your legal fees could be astronomical!

Even if legal, the specifics of using marijuana vary from state to state. Maine has a wonderfully flexible law allowing the possession of up to 2.5 ounces of finished, prepared marijuana. It allows the certified patient to grow their own – up to six mature plants – and allows licensed growers (called "caregivers") to grow marijuana for patients. The caregiver arrangement means that growing marijuana is not a monopoly of a few large corporations – and becoming a caregiver has become a widespread cottage industry in the state. It also means that many of those who have honed their skills at cultivating this plant over the past few years (or decades) are now able to convert those skills into a marketable commodity! The availability of options other than a dispensary for obtaining medical marijuana means competition in the marketplace. While dispensaries charge $300 to $400 per ounce, caregivers often charge half that.

And for those who cannot afford even the costs from a caregiver, growing your own becomes an option. The big challenge of course, especially in a cold climate like that of Maine, is that posed by trying to grow enough marijuana in the summer growing season to last all year. And the obvious question is: how can you grow six mature plants if you are only allowed to possess 2.5 ounces of marijuana? Unless you are a very bad gardener, given that a healthy marijuana plant should yield three to five ounces of useful marijuana, you would be violating the law with those six mature plants! The Maine law takes all of that into consideration. You are actually allowed up to eight pounds of harvested marijuana – as long as it is not trimmed, cleaned, or otherwise processed for use. You are also allowed "any number" of seedlings – this is referred to as an "incidental" amount of marijuana. So you can plant twenty or thirty seeds, as long as you start thinning out the stragglers and the male plants as they grow, leaving you with only six maturing plants.

"Where do I get seeds" I am asked frequently. I don't think Burpee's has the seeds you need, and Home Depot doesn't stock them. Often patients get seeds from other patients that they know, or even from caregivers. Cuttings, or "clones", are often shared among caregivers. I have other patients tell me that they order their seeds either online or from ads in the back of magazines such as "High Times". Surprisingly, even though this is not legal, most people get their seeds as ordered. One patient recently advised me that he had ordered seeds, never to see his seeds or money again. What a fantastic scam these "sellers" have – what is the duped customer going to do – complain to the authorities? So I advise people who want to order online to try to get a friend's referral for a reliable source.

There are other aspects of medical marijuana laws in various states that may be important. In our state, the law specifically protects a certified patient from arrest for possession of the "paraphernalia" necessary for the use of medical marijuana. It also protects certified medical marijuana patient renters from being evicted by their landlords for the legal smoking of marijuana in a rental apartment or home – with the exception that an apartment building that is designated as "non-smoking" can remain just that – legal to use medical marijuana if you are certified – just not legal to smoke it! Likewise no protection is offered for those who feel they must smoke their medical marijuana in a non-smoking hotel room.

In NO state does a medical marijuana law protect you from being arrested for DUI/OUI/DWI. But of course, law enforcement does not have the same tools as they do for DUI arrests involving alcohol. No "breathalyzer", no blood level testing, etc. Many have suggested such testing be developed, but the problem is that levels of actual impairment vary a great deal with any given level of marijuana – someone who is a daily user of marijuana may function fairly well at a given level, where a casual user may be significantly impaired at that same level. The definition of "impaired" when it comes to drugs other than alcohol rests mainly on a driver's performance on the field sobriety test – if you are stopped for driving erratically, will you be able to walk heel-to-toe and touch your finger to your nose? If not, you will be arrested – whether you have used any drug or not! I often have patients with disabilities tell me that they doubt that they could pass a field sobriety test even on their most stone-cold-sober days. My only advice is to not to let themselves be in a position to be asked to do a field sobriety test. Otherwise they will find themselves in front of a judge trying to convince them that the video being seen of staggering and falling is not an indication of a lack of sobriety. The judge has heard that story already twenty tines that day, so good luck with that!

Obviously you do not want to get stoned and drive. You also do not want to get stoned and work with your table saw or climb up on the roof to repair that leaking hole. Common sense and responsibility are the keys to using medical marijuana. But also – discretion is important as well. You do not need to advertise to the world that you are using medical marijuana. If you are on your way home from the dispensary with a baggie full of marijuana sitting in plain sight on your passenger seat and you get pulled over for coasting through the stop sign, your stop is going to be a bit more complicated than had you put your new purchase out of sight. And while the law might protect you from an arrest for possession if you light up in public, you can be arrested for disturbing the peace any time you are being an ass in public. So be cool...

The illegal nature of marijuana at the federal level continues to cause trouble for those wishing to use it legally, however. Obviously the physicians at the VA medical centers and clinics will not certify their patients – many are unwilling to even discuss it, even though it is - in almost half the states - now the drug of choice for treating PTSD. Overall in Maine *only 3% of physicians* are willing to provide medical marijuana certification to their patients. At all levels the bureaucrats have sent down the message: "do not certify your patients for medical marijuana". Maine, being a poor and largely rural state, has many rural health clinics and community health centers which receive federal support. The bureaucrats live in perpetual fear that medical marijuana certification would result in their loss of federal support. But even some of the large health centers such as Eastern Maine Medical Center in Bangor have advised their medical staff to refrain from providing the legal means to use this safe and effective plant medicine. It causes me great shame for my profession that even our local cancer specialists – whose patients are often riddled with cancer and who then get pumped full of some of the most toxic chemicals known to man – refuse to offer the benefits of this plant medicine – this weed – to those patients!

Can I be fired if I am legally using marijuana?

In a word: yes! I am not aware of any state which protects you from being fired for using medical marijuana. I always advise patients that if they have a job which requires them to pee in a cup either randomly or for cause, that they should not use medical marijuana. What if you are a school bus driver and wish to use a little medical marijuana to help your pain at bedtime – or even just on weekend nights? If you are involved in an accident and THC shows up in your urine – and it may show up in your urine several weeks after your last use – at worst you could face criminal prosecution and at best the newspapers would label you as a "dope-crazed impaired bus driver hell-bent on endangering the lives of children". Even if the accident had nothing to do with your actions you might suffer permanent repercussions. I have a patient who works periodically on scheduled repairs at nuclear plants. He always has to pee in a cup before starting a job, but his jobs are all scheduled well in advance, so he knows to stop using his medical marijuana weeks before the beginning of any new job. But I think he is playing with fire – a positive test would mean he would be out of a job and probably disqualified for any work of this nature in the future. Sadly, he would be better off (legally, anyway) by using oxycodone for his pain!

You may think that your employer will allow a positive THC finding on your pee test, but there are no guarantees. And if a company is looking for any reason to downsize – or if your boss doesn't like you – your pee test may give them a reason to tell you goodbye.

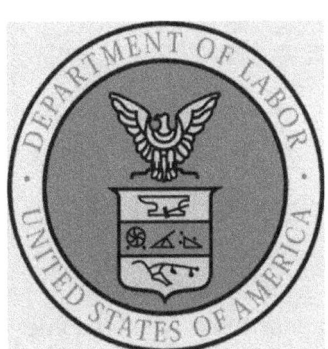

And many workplaces participate in the U.S. Department of Labor's "Drug Free Workplace" program. Any company that contracts with the U.S. Government is supposed to provide a drug-free workplace for their employees. And since marijuana is illegal for any and all purposes at the federal level, that means medical marijuana as well.

I find it amusing and ironic that the State of Maine requires medical marijuana dispensaries to be "drug-free workplaces"!

Do THEY allow their employees to use legal medical marijuana?

Chapter 3: What happens when I register?

Every state has its own mechanism for certifying or registering medical marijuana users. Maine has an interesting history in this aspect – Maine's medical marijuana program was passed by a largely Republican, conservative legislature. In New England conservatism is often of the libertarian variety. The legislators felt that it was not the government's role to prevent adults from using a medicinal plant – a weed – for those purposes for which it had proven to be useful. When the law was passed and the Maine Department of Health and Human Services was charged with implementing it, they decided to require certified patients to register with Maine DHHS.

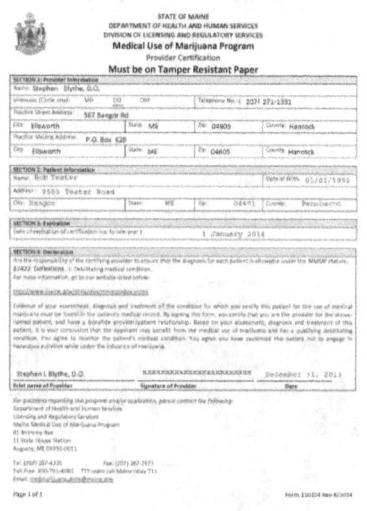

The process created was that after getting the certificate signed by the physician, the patient would send a copy with $100 to DHHS and then receive a "card" which made them legal. The legislators were very unhappy with this – it was not their intent that a person legally using this medicinal plant be required to register with the government. So they rewrote that section of the law specifically saying that patients did NOT have to register with DHHS. They kept the option of registering for those who for some reason preferred the little laminated card – but insisted that this process be without charge to the patient. Most of my patients opt not to register with the government.

This system did leave the DHHS in a quandary. For years they had no idea how many patients were being certified and where they lived, and had no idea which physicians were doing the certification.

Medical Marijuana

This would be useful information to have – there have been a number of abuses of the system by charlatans intent on making a quick buck and by people who should not have been certifying patients in the first place. For example, an out-of-state physician's assistant set up shop in Bangor and certified lots of patients, signing a physician's name to the certificates. PA's are not allowed to certify patients in Maine – and in this case the physician whose name was being used apparently had no knowledge that this was being done. When DHHS found out about this, the PA left the state before he could be prosecuted – but the dispensaries all received letters informing them that these certificates were not valid. So I have certified a number of patients who had paid $250 for a worthless piece of paper!

The state of Maine has now changed their program for certification. Physicians (or now nurse practitioners as well) who wish to certify patients must register with an on-line program. They must then order special paper from DHHS. When a patient is in the office and has met the requirements for certification, the physician/NP logs on, enters basic demographic data on the patient, and prints out a card for them. DHHS swears they do not maintain records of patient names – only the demographic information. I look forward to seeing the 2015 annual report next year with the information gathered from this system.

Other states are not so patient-friendly. Many states require patients to register with the state. The referendum which was recently defeated in Florida (60% of the vote required to pass – it only received 58%) would have required patients to register with the state. This situation raises a great deal of concern with me, especially if there are no clearly stated guidelines for what happens to that information. Does law enforcement have access to it? What about patients who are employed by the state – teachers, DOT workers, etc.? Do their employers have access to that information? What about professionals who are licensed by the state – from hairdressers to plumbers to counselors to brain surgeons? Do their licensing boards have access to that information? While I have a reasonable amount of concern about brain surgeons using medical marijuana, I assume that a professional can be just as professional about the responsible and safe use of marijuana as they can be about the use of alcohol.

Chapter 4: What conditions does medical marijuana treat?

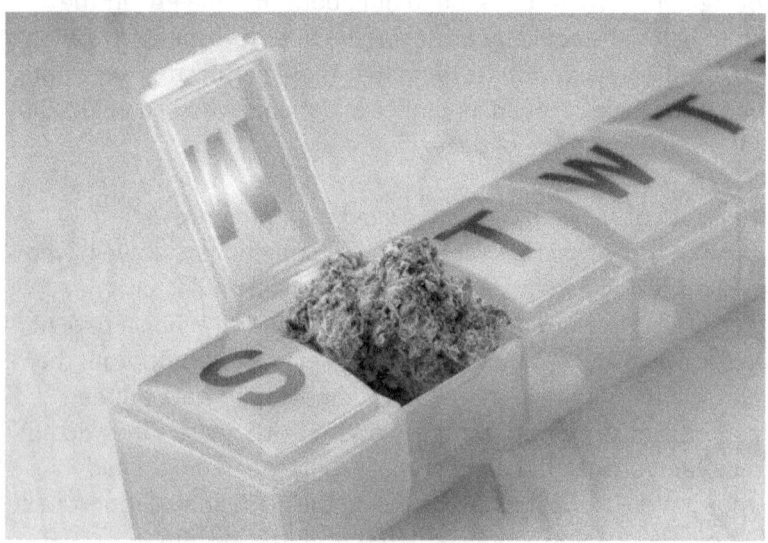

Will a bud a day keep the doctor away?

States that allow medical marijuana vary in terms of what conditions may be treated. Some states leave it to the discretion of the certifying physician. Others, such as Maine, have a specific list of qualifying conditions. Unfortunately, the list is carved in stone, and although there exists a mechanism for adding conditions to the list, the ultimate decision to do so rests with the Director of the Department of Health and Human Services, who is against the program, and can deny the addition of conditions to the list by saying that "marijuana has not been proven safe and effective in the treatment of said condition". No kidding – it is not like anyone in the United States CAN study the safety and effectiveness of marijuana. I petitioned the Maine DHHS this past year to add Obsessive-Compulsive Disorder to the list. We had hearings where patients and physicians testified, and some patients presented written testimony. All to no avail, because marijuana "has not been proven safe and effective for treating OCD". I was disappointed but not surprised.

PAIN: I list pain first for a very good reason. Pain is the reason that 90% of my patients seek certification to use medical marijuana. Marijuana is useful for those with chronic pain – and we generally do a piss-poor job of treating our patients with pain. We have few tools in our tool chest for treating pain.

Opioids remain the only really useful prescription drug for treatment of pain. But the use of opioids is rife with conflict, complication, and controversy.

A Note on Terminology:

"Narcotic"	Any chemical, including alcohol, which can produce euphoria, stupor, or somnolence. In legal terminology "narcotic" refers to any illegal controlled substance, even stimulants such as amphetamine. The use of the term "narcotic" to refer to pain medication is overbroad and outdated and is now discouraged.
"Opiate"	Medications derived from the opium poppy such as opium, morphine, and codeine. Technically only applies to the naturally-derived drugs.
"Opioid"	Any medication, whether natural or synthetic, which acts on the opiate receptors in the body. This includes synthetics such as fentanyl, methadone, and others. This is now the preferred term for pain medications that act on the opiate receptors in the body.

Medical Marijuana

The conflicts and controversies surrounding the use of opioids are because of their potential complications – both short-term and long-term.

Opioids are addictive. Everyone knows that. This makes them a less-than-ideal medication for chronic use. But the addictive nature of these drugs has made it sometimes impossible for pain patients to get their pain treated. Even as recently as the 1940's the AMA published position papers stating that terminal cancer patients should not have their pain treated with opioids for fear of addiction!

I was recently at a pain medicine conference, and one of the speakers made the statement: "There is no role for opioid medications in the treatment of chronic back pain". My first thought was: "Good for him – he has never experienced pain". The next speaker to take the podium was bristling with anger when he got up. He said:

> Our role as physicians is to heal or to cure our patients whenever possible. But sometimes that is not possible, and our role then becomes to relieve their suffering. And we must use every tool at our disposal to do that.

I am totally in agreement with this statement – and marijuana is not a miracle drug for pain treatment – but it is another tool in our small toolbox of pain treatment options.

Patients who use opioid medications on a regular basis - to the point where it is in their body all of the time - are very likely to become addicted. I try to encourage patients to use short-acting opioids such as hydrocodone and oxycodone at most twice a day, since these medications stay in the body five or six hours only. This makes it less likely to create an addiction. Patients who have conditions which put them in misery 24 hours a day simply have to accept addiction as a consequence of their treatment. Studies have shown that most people (but clearly not all) who undergo an effective treatment of their painful condition (such as surgery) can successfully stop their opioid medication. For some it is not easy.

FYI: "Oxycontin®" is a brand-name long-acting form of the opioid medication oxycodone. Many confuse the two. While Oxycontin® is oxycodone, oxycodone is not necessarily Oxycontin®!

The other big problem with the chronic use of opioid medications is the development of tolerance. Opioids block the "pain receptors" in the body. This helps – but the body is pretty smart and makes *more* pain receptors! With most opioid medications, after a few months of constant use the effectiveness starts to lessen and a higher dose is required to block the pain. This seems to be a relentless cycle – I have a few patients on massive doses of oxycodone who continue to have constant severe pain.

The other interesting fact about the increase in pain receptors is a greater sensitivity to pain. I see patients on large doses of opioids for their chronic pain who suffer something like a sprained ankle and come to the office crying like a baby, requesting even more medication for their pain! My first thought is that this is something that most of us would treat with some ice and ibuprofen – but these patients may actually be having more pain than the rest of us would suffer with the same injury.

The other most worrisome thing about opioids is that they suppress breathing, especially if combined with any other sedative, including alcohol. For this reason, anyone who takes a little more than prescribed, especially if mixed with a tranquilizer or sleeping pill and a little alcohol, may go to sleep and never wake up. Accidental overdoses are not rare with these medications – as many as 16,000 Americans die each year from accidental overdose. The worst of these for this effect is methadone – it is a cheap and useful long-acting medication for chronic pain. Long-acting oxycodone may cost $300 or more per month – methadone costs a small fraction of that. But the problem with methadone is that while it takes a few days for the pain relieving effect to reach a plateau, the depressing effect on breathing continues to increase for seven or eight days or so. For that reason the dose should not be increased more often than every ten days. But the impatient patient who ups their dose sooner than this may find themselves no longer in pain...forever. I have read statistics that say that while only 5% of pain patients in the US are prescribed methadone for their pain, this drug accounts for almost one-third of the accidental overdose deaths from opioids.

But marijuana, which kills no one, is apparently the truly evil drug:

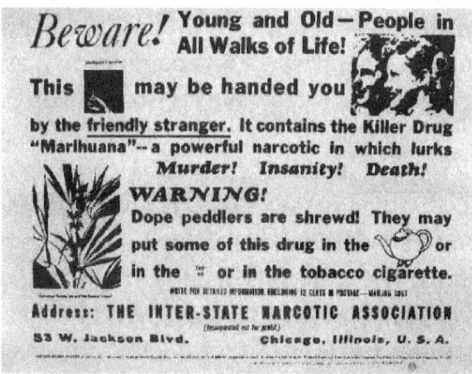

The bitter irony is that methadone is less likely to generate the tolerance seen with the other opioids. I do not start pain patients on methadone but I have several that I have inherited from other physicians who have retired or relocated. These patients have been on the same dose of methadone for their pain for many years without requiring an increase in dose.

I have read articles that blame "loose" prescribing of opioid medications for an increase in suicides by overdose. I resent this assertion. The suicide rate nationally has gone down dramatically since the advent of newer classes of antidepressant medications. What has happened also is that the percentage of suicides by firearm has dropped and the percentage of suicides by overdose has increased. I have to think that if given the choice, most people would prefer the more peaceful exit afforded by an opioid overdose unless they were really, really angry at those they were leaving behind.

Another side benefit, if you will, of "loose" prescribing of prescription pain medication is the more widespread availability of pharmaceutical-grade opioids to those who would abuse them. This sounds like a bad thing, but recently the State of Maine tightened up their coverage of pain medications obtained through "MaineCare", the state's Medicaid program. The result was a sudden increase in overdose deaths from cheaper heroin – whose variable purity always makes shooting up a game of Russian roulette.

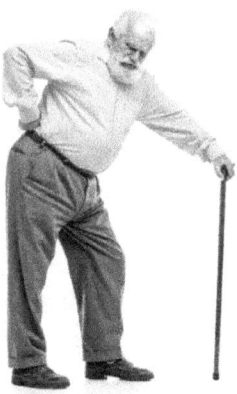

The typical patient that I certify for medical marijuana is seeking relief from chronic pain, and the average age is about 55.

I also like to remind those critics of rational prescribing of pain medication that chronic untreated or under-treated pain IS a major cause of suicide. An example is George Eastman – founder of the Eastman-Kodak company. There was a time when any photograph taken meant sending the film (if not the camera itself) to the Eastman-Kodak Company for processing. All movies proclaimed that they were in "Eastman Color". George Eastman, though, in his later years developed spinal stenosis which resulted in intense back pain. In spite of being one of the richest men on the planet, in 1932 he put a bullet through his heart. He left a note saying: "Why wait"? Even for George Eastman life was not worth living.

The other HUGE problem with opioid medications is that they take away pain – both physical and *mental* pain. They make people feel good. And if you put them quickly in to your blood stream by snorting them up your nose or injecting them directly, you can feel REALLY good – at least for a while. Then pretty soon you feel like crap unless you are using the drug. This makes them a much sought-after medication. As a physician I have no tool for measuring whether someone is really in pain, and if so how much pain they are really suffering. So is the patient seeking drugs – or simply seeking relief from their pain? I really don't know. This makes treating pain patients a – well, a pain. I would not be surprised if 10% of my pain patients are misusing, abusing, or misdirecting their medications. I fire any patients that are clearly misusing their medications – if they try to get opioids from multiple physicians, if they frequently "lose" their medication or have their medication stolen, if they frequently demand early refills, or if they use other drugs of abuse (such as crystal meth, heroin, methadone, cocaine, etc.). But what this means is that I and other physicians who are willing to do pain management are forced to treat our pain patients as drug-seekers. We make them pee in a cup on a regular (or irregular and random) basis and we sometimes make them come in at unscheduled intervals and bring their pills for a pill-count. We are forced to look with a skeptical eye any time a patient requests a higher dose or a more frequent use of their medication – again: are they "drug-seeking" or seeking relief? I have no way of knowing.

One of the things I like about offering medical marijuana for sufferers of chronic pain is the fact that *the patient* is in control of their treatment: no one is looking over their shoulder counting pills and scolding them for how much medicine they are using.

Medical Marijuana

So – all of this is just to summarize that we have pretty lousy tools for treating pain. There are some other medications – Lyrica and gabapentin which may help nerve pain, and Cymbalta® (duloxetine) which may help mild pain and helps the depression associated with chronic pain. There is definitely physical therapy, which is a must for many patients. There are electrical stimulators – from TENS units applied to the skin to spinal cord stimulators implanted surgically. But there is nothing that simply takes away the pain like the opioids.

Then along comes medical marijuana for pain. Of my medical marijuana patients who use it for pain almost all feel that it is a very helpful tool. Most of them tell me the same thing: "It doesn't make the pain go away, but it lets me put the pain in the back of my mind and do what I need to do – or it lets me ignore the pain and go to sleep". For a medication that is neither addictive nor going to kill you, that is a pretty good thing! Marijuana does not suppress breathing, even when combined with opioids, alcohol, or tranquilizers. It doesn't cause a physical addiction. It generally does not seem to cause a tolerance.

It is unfortunate that a small percentage of pain patients are advised by their pain care providers that they will no longer be prescribed opioid medications if they become certified and try medical marijuana. I think this is really sad – they are clearly different tools used differently. (In my mind this would be like going to the hardware store for a screwdriver and being told that you have to turn in your hammer before you can get a screwdriver!) And most of my patients who use marijuana to treat their pain are only interested in using it in the evening and at bedtime – they have no interest in possibly being "stoned" in the daytime when they have to drive or go to work.

One last point: in an article published in the Journal of the American Medical Association: Internal Medicine (2014:174 (10):1668-1673) Dr. Marcus Bachhuber and colleagues reported on their study that showed that when states enacted medical marijuana laws the rate of opioid overdose deaths decreased by an average of almost 25% and by the sixth year of medical marijuana the overdose rate was down by one-third! This study could not determine the cause of this decline – but possibilities include patients having better quality of life due to better control of their pain and beneficial effects on depression from medical marijuana.

PTSD: Most of us in my generation have friends and family members who were sent to Vietnam to fight in the swamps. No matter what side of this conflict you were on, no one could deny that it was a war more terrible on the individual soldier than any we had fought before. Wading through swamp and jungle in search of an enemy that could not be identified – the "enemy" and the "friendlies" looked identical. Until someone shot your comrade or threw a grenade at you, you couldn't know. Millions of young men returned from that conflict to suffer from "flashbacks" – terrible nightmares that interfered with sleep, and daytime images that inserted themselves in the thoughts whenever certain triggers (such as the sound of a car backfiring) were encountered. Many of these veterans discovered that the only way they could keep the "flashbacks" away was to use marijuana. We now call this post-traumatic stress disorder, or PTSD. We see it in many of those who have survived trauma – not just the trauma of combat, but the trauma of serious accidents and physical and/or sexual assault.

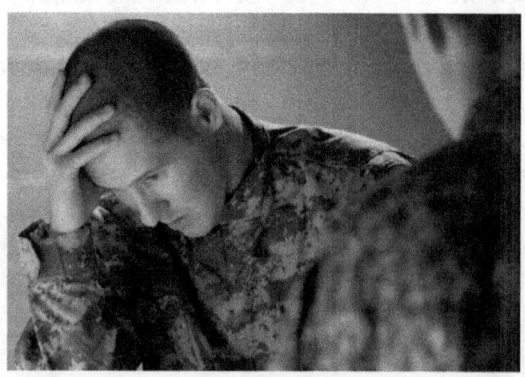

Medical Marijuana

It is now widely acknowledged that marijuana is an effective treatment for PTSD. My patients who are veterans ALL tell me the same thing: "it is far better than anything the VA has ever prescribed for me". And those prescriptions have included Effexor, Prozac, Zoloft, Zyprexa, Abilify, Seroquel – you name it.

The Israelis have studied marijuana for the treatment of PTSD for a number of years now. They have even developed an animal model for PTSD: rats that are living in cages with metal screen floors are randomly subjected to electrical shocks after a loud bell rings. Pretty soon the rats display signs of stress, and the "trigger" of a loud bell causes a response just as if they had been shocked again. Treatment with marijuana demonstrates its benefit for these poor rats.

Anxiety is often treated with marijuana. It is one of the most commonly used self-medication agents for this. Indeed, marijuana at very low levels may help with anxiety, although higher amounts are often associated with increased anxiety, agitation, or paranoia. Those treating their anxiety with marijuana need to be

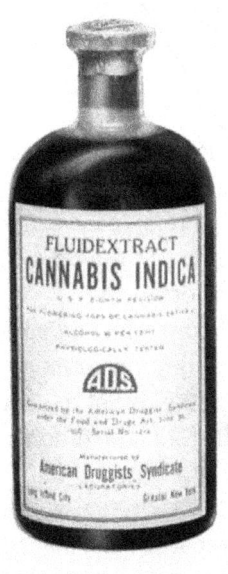

careful and need to realize that just because a little bit helps doesn't mean that more will be more helpful. Some states recognize anxiety as a condition which can be treated by medical marijuana. Maine does not – I suspect that the crafters of the law felt that the diagnosis of anxiety would be the entryway for anyone seeking the legal use of marijuana to get certified. After all, who doesn't have some anxiety every now and then? The anxiety associated with bipolar disorder may also be effectively treated with marijuana, but in these patients there is probably an even greater risk of agitation or paranoia.

Medical Marijuana

Inflammatory Bowel Disease is a collection of diseases which cause the intestines to be inflamed, resulting in diarrhea – often bloody, often painful, and frequently life-altering. This name applies to Crohn's Disease and ulcerative colitis/proctitis, and can include others such as chronic *C. dificile* colitis. The colon contains a large number of endocannabinoid receptors – the natural receptors which are stimulated by both compounds in our bodies as well as cannabinoids from marijuana. I have had a number of such patients who have had dramatic benefit from medical marijuana. One patient, as an example, tells me that he had used marijuana illegally for five years. His Crohn's Disease causes him to wake each morning with abdominal pain and nausea, and with no appetite. Within ten minutes of taking a hit of marijuana he feels fine, and is able to eat. I asked him if this caused him any problems – did he end up getting stoned in the morning before going to work? His answer was: "Oh hell no – I roll joints and I take just one hit and put it out – a joint lasts me a week"! This medicine has allowed him to lead a normal life in spite of his disease. Anyone with inflammatory bowel disease needs to be under the care of a gastroenterologist as well as using medical marijuana. Without close monitoring and intervention when needed these conditions can cause bowel perforation and even death.

Muscle spasm caused by underlying neuromuscular diseases such as cerebral palsy or MS may respond very well to medical marijuana. There are many prescription muscle relaxers available as well, so a patient with muscle spasms must weigh the side effects and usefulness of all of their options. Most of the prescription muscle relaxers do not cause a "stoned feeling" (although some do in some patients) but all commonly cause drowsiness which may be debilitating. As with the use of medical marijuana for pain, many patients reserve this for night-time use if the dose required to help causes too much of a buzz.

Nausea and anorexia (loss of appetite) accompany many chronic diseases and are commonly encountered as side effects of chemotherapy. This is the major use for prescription THC, or dronabinol. Dronabinal (generic Marinol®) has the advantages of clear-cut dosing and coverage by insurance companies, but many people feel that the whole marijuana, especially when custom-dosed by smoking or vaping, works better.

Hepatitis C is on the list of qualifying conditions in Maine. This is interesting, because there is no discussion that the patient actually must be *sick* with Hepatitis C – just that they have it. Although Maine has not legalized the recreational use of medical marijuana for the general public, they essentially have given the OK for this population. The obvious reason is that if these patients want to get high, alcohol would be a very poor choice. Patients with Hepatitis C who drink may quickly end up on the liver transplant list, where those who do not drink may never. If you have liver failure you almost always end up disabled and poor – meaning that the state ends up paying a large part of your transplantation expenses! They don't want THAT! So they want you to PLEASE smoke marijuana instead of drinking!

One interesting caveat: there are **two important blood tests** for determining whether or not someone has Hepatitis C, and many patients and even many health care providers do not seem to be clear on this. I have had several patients referred for certification on the basis of having Hepatitis C when in fact they did not have it. I just had to tell a patient this week as I write this that I had "good news and bad news". The bad news of course was that they were not qualified to be certified for medical marijuana – the really good news was that they *did not have Hepatitis C* in spite of what they had been told.

The first test for Hepatitis C is the "antibody test". This shows whether or not you have ever been exposed to the virus. When that happens your body produces antibodies to fight of the infection. Most people do not totally fight off the virus, and they maintain a low-level infection for the rest of their lives (unless they are successfully treated). The second blood test is the "viral load" test (also called the RNA test or the PCR test). This actually looks for genetic material from Hepatitis C virus in the bloodstream. About one out of every eight people who are exposed to the virus fight off the virus and cure themselves of the disease. So having a positive antibody test but a negative RNA or viral load test means that you were exposed – but you do NOT have the disease! So – "sorry".

OCD is the abbreviation for obsessive-compulsive disorder, the most common of which is probably nail-biting. Hair twirling is also common. But OCD can take severe life-altering manifestations. Some people have such severe hair-twirling (called trichotillomania) that they leave themselves bald. Others have a skin-picking disorder called dermatotillomania where they constantly pick holes in their skin. Others cut themselves. Others have obsessions about hygiene, and others have counting obsessions where they have to count things, they have a special number which they obsess about, or they tap or touch things a specific number of times. Someone with a tapping OCD, for example, might not be able to leave their room until they have made multiple trips around the room, touching or tapping everything six times. Someone with a hygiene OCD may spend an hour brushing their teeth – resulting in damage to their enamel. I have a patient who is a kleptomaniac (another OCD) who has an obsession with spoons as well as with the number four. What this means is that whenever she is someplace where she has the opportunity she will steal four spoons. She must have quite a collection! I have tried working with her in a behavioral approach, suggesting that she never leave her home without taking four of her favorite spoons with her. This seems like a funny obsession – at least until she gets arrested.

OCD is extremely difficult to treat. You cannot talk someone out of an obsession. Sometimes these patients will respond to the common antidepressants, but often it requires very high doses. I had a patient in the past with severe disfiguring skin-picking who had no response even from 80mg of Prozac. He ended up taking an anti-psychotic medication which stopped his obsession but probably lowered his IQ by 20 points and made him rather zombie-like in his affect. But he stopped picking, by golly! There are limited studies showing that synthetic THC (sold as the prescription drug Marinol©) can be somewhat helpful in the treatment of OCD. Some patients with OCD have benefitted greatly from medical marijuana. The most extreme example of a patient of mine with OCD helped by medical marijuana was a young woman who had a hygiene obsession. Her mother was along with her for her visit, and the young woman explained how she spent four hours a day in the shower. Her mother laughingly talked about their needing to buy the largest hot-water tank available. When this young woman started using marijuana for her PTSD her OCD improved dramatically. "I can take a shower like a normal person" she said. In addition, she told me that her grades in her college chemistry class went from a "D" to an "A". She told me:

> *Before using the marijuana I could not get through a homework assignment or test – I would think about the question, think of an answer, rethink the question, think about whether or not my answer was right, and just not be able to get through it. Now I can look at the question, write down the answer, and move on to the next question.*

Unfortunately, in spite of my petition to the Maine DHHS to add OCD to the list of qualifying conditions, the Director refused to consider it, so patients without other qualifying disorders cannot legally benefit from this plant medicine.

Other uses: reports of uses of marijuana for other purposes ranging from HIV to treating cancer have been reported. If scientists and physicians in the United States would be allowed to research this plant we would know for sure what is fact and what is fancy.

Chapter 5: How to use marijuana

The classic way to use marijuana is to smoke it. In one sense smoking is the perfect drug delivery system: you inhale the medicine, it goes into the blood stream right away, and within minutes you know how it is working and if you have the right dose. No waiting around for an hour – like with a pill – to see what effect it will have. Smoking can be with a traditional marijuana cigarette – a "joint" or a "blunt". It can also be done with a water-pipe which cools the smoke and is less likely to trigger coughing, or with a "bong", a pipe with a large chamber which allows the smoke to cool before the large quantity is inhaled into the lungs.

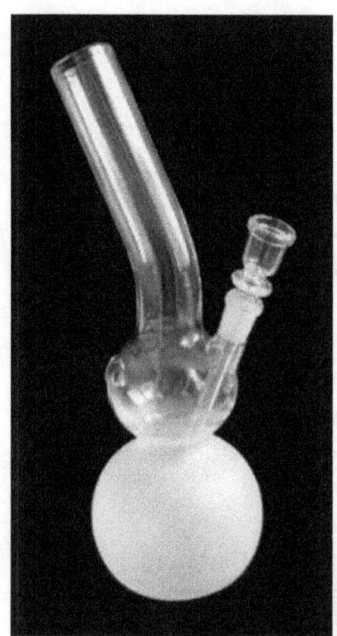

A bong is used by sucking on the mouthpiece (at the top of the bong shown here) while a finger is held over the carburation port until the chamber fills with smoke. At that point the finger is withdrawn, opening the port, and the cooled smoke in the chamber is inhaled into the lungs.

Obviously inhaling smoke into the lungs is not the best thing for our health. Smoking marijuana can trigger coughing paroxysms and could trigger a severe asthma attack or exacerbation of COPD in those affected. It is unknown whether or not smoking marijuana can lead to lung cancer. Undoubtedly there are carcinogens in most smoke – but cigarette smokers who get lung cancer have often smoked 1 or 2 packs per day – 20 to 40 cigarettes per day – for many years. Very few marijuana smokers smoke that much!

One alternative to smoking is to use a vaporizer. <u>This is not your grandmother's vaporizer!</u> A vaporizer, or a "vape", is a device designed to heat up the marijuana to about 380 degrees – hot enough to evaporate the THC and CBD but not hot enough to ignite the marijuana material. So although the result is a hot vapor that is inhaled, it is not smoke. So it is probably safer. It also has other benefits. A small portable vape such as the Pax® is very discrete. One of my patients runs a small store. He has chronic back pain, and he tells me:

> When my back pain acts up, I can't really go out back and smoke, because then I get bloodshot eyes and I smell like I just smoked a joint. But I can go out back and vape, and my eyes don't get red, I don't smell, and no one looks at me funny.

Vaping does produce an odor, but it is not nearly as strong as that produced by burning the marijuana in a joint or a pipe. Some people find the vapor just as irritating as smoke. Some feel the results from vaping equal the results of smoking, but others tell me they do not think it works as well.

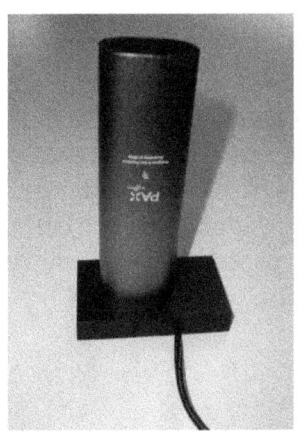

A "PAX®" vaporizer sitting in its charging stand. This is a very popular vape which is fairly expensive. It is all stainless steel construction, very solid, and comes with a 10-year warranty. The folks at the local dispensary tell me that if ever a customer has a problem with their unit the customer service is excellent.

Medical Marijuana

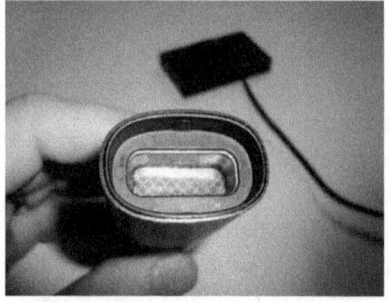 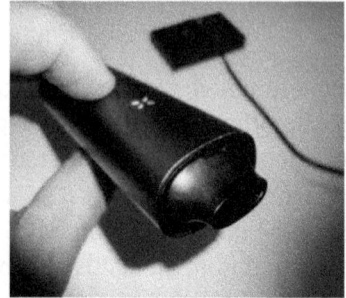

One end of the Pax® has the marijuana holding chamber with a magnetic lid. The other end is the mouthpiece – it pops out when pressed, which turns the unit on. A small light on the side turns green when 380 degrees is reached. It cleans easily with a cotton swab, a pipe cleaner, and a little rubbing alcohol.

How expensive is a vaporizer? My local dispensary sells them from $80 to $600 – "depending upon how fancy you want and how much money you have". They like the mid-range units, which seem to be well made and come with good warrantees. They tell me those companies have good reputations for having good products and good customer service. On the other hand, one patient recently told me he bought a vape unit for $25 at a head shop. "When it breaks, I'll buy another one" he said.

A Hash Oil Pen Vaporizer is the latest trendy mechanism for using marijuana. These look and act like an electronic cigarette. Our local dispensary (in Ellsworth) is for now the only one in the State of Maine to carry this – because things like hash oil cannot be shipped across state lines, they contracted with the company in Colorado to send an employee along with necessary equipment to Maine to produce the hash oil cartridges for their customers.

Medical Marijuana

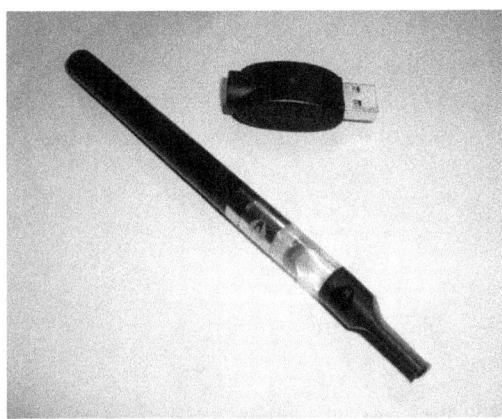

This is the "O-Pen Vape®", now available in Maine.

At the top is the charger, which plugs into a USB cell phone charger or the USB port of a computer.

The charge usually lasts through one whole cartridge – about 70 "hits". Most patients find that one or two hits is a sufficient dose. The pen vape produces no smoke and very little odor. It is discrete – anyone who saw you use it would think you were using an e-cigarette. Even the tip glows when you inhale on it, just like an e-cig.

There are several great things about the pen vape. The first is that there is no flame or ash involved. If you awake with pain at 3 AM, you can reach over to your bedside table, pick this up, take a dose, and return to sleep without even turning on a light! It is undoubtedly safer than breathing in smoke. AND – it is very inexpensive! The hash oil can be made from leaf which is normally not used for smoking. A cartridge runs about $20 – which as stated, is enough for 35 to 70 doses. THAT is cheap! The pen itself runs about $25. It can be purchased online, along with empty cartridges, if you are inclined to make your own hash oil. Just don't use the butane extraction technique – many people in Colorado get seriously injured every year doing this.
The only negative about the pen vape is that you do not have the choice of strains as you do with buying the plant for smoking or vaping. The hash oil comes as "sativa" or "indica".

Medical Marijuana

Edibles is the common term for any form of marijuana that is made to be ingested through the mouth. Many dispensaries sell large amounts of edibles, and many patients make their own. It is very, very important to be informed about the pros and cons of edibles before using them.

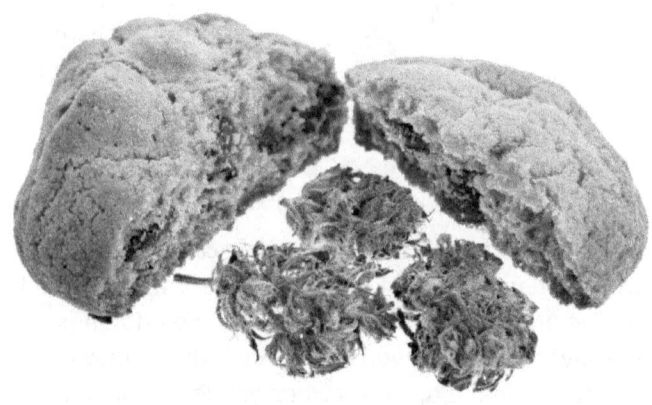

There are pros and cons about ingesting marijuana. Many prefer edibles, either for the effect or because they want to stay away from smoking. When marijuana is ingested, it has to be digested – the plant material has to be broken down by stomach acid and digestive enzymes. The THC, CBD, and other compounds are then absorbed through the wall of the small intestine into the bloodstream around the intestines (called the "portal system"). This blood is processed in the liver before heading out to the body. Some people feel that ingested marijuana is better for "body effect" – especially for pain and inflammation, whereas smoked marijuana is better when a "head effect" is wanted. But timing is everything, and ingested marijuana has different timing than smoked or vaped marijuana.

Smoking or vaping is in some ways the ideal drug delivery system – the drug goes into your bloodstream right away, and within minutes you know how it is working – and whether or not you need another dose. Not like taking a pill and waiting an hour to see how you feel. But ingesting marijuana is more like that pill – it can take up to an hour or longer for ingested marijuana to work – depending on what other food is in the GI tract and the type of food that the marijuana was mixed in. The good news about timing is that the effect may last up to eight hours (as opposed to 3-4 hours from smoking). This makes it useful for bedtime use for pain or PTSD.

But if patience is not a virtue you possess, edibles can land you in BIG trouble. In the spring of 2014 a young man fell to his death from his hotel balcony in Denver. He and a buddy had traveled to Colorado for spring break to experience the legal marijuana. I heard this story on the news and immediately looked at my wife and said: "I bet they got cookies". Sure enough, the next day when more information became available, that is what happened. And you can just picture the scene: two kids sitting around their hotel room. They have just returned from the dispensary with their goody bag. Maybe they are eating a pizza and having a few beers. They eat a cookie. After fifteen minutes or so, one remarks how he is not feeling anything. Perhaps the cookies are not very strong – so they have another. Then perhaps after another fifteen or twenty minutes they get impatient and decide to have another. Who knows how much marijuana he ingested? It is very rare for someone to smoke weed and get so confused or stupid that they fall off a balcony.

Dosing is therefore the HUGE problem with edibles. If you smoke or vape, you take your time and you figure out when to stop. It is not rocket science, and there is no guess work. But if you are eating an edible, you won't know for up to an hour or so how it will work. The other problem is knowing from the start what the dose within the edible actually is.

I always discuss this in a medical marijuana consultation. I point out that the local dispensary, which houses a state-licensed kitchen, makes and sells these great big cookies. "So is this cookie a dose?", I asked at a recent visit. "Oh, no!" I was advised. "A pinch of cookie, or at most a fourth of the cookie, is a dose". Very often when I mention this the patient's eyes will get real big, and they will say: "Well that explains THAT!" and then they go on to tell me almost the story, which almost always goes like: "My boyfriend gave me a cookie that he bought at the dispensary and I ate the whole thing. I slept for three days!"

Back when I went to college, if someone made marijuana brownies or cookies they did it by crumbling up their marijuana leaves in the cookie dough. It didn't taste bad, but eating it felt like someone had put hay in your brownies. These days marijuana is infused in warm vegetable oil or butter which is then later used to make the edibles. How strong is the oil? Who knows? It depends upon the recipe, the amount of marijuana used, the strength of the marijuana used, and any other variables such as the temperature and duration of the infusion. Some recipes call for freezing the marijuana before infusing it in the oil, with the thought that it breaks down the plant cells and increases the extraction. The result is that you may have no clue about the dose of marijuana in the edibles you buy at the dispensary!

The Denver Post did a study in the fall of 2014 looking at this issue. In Colorado the dispensaries label their edibles with content of THC. A normal dose is considered to be 10mg. The Denver Post took samples of edibles from numerous dispensaries and analyzed them for THC content. One dispensary was selling "edibles" with no THC in them! But the edibles from the other dispensaries, which were supposed to contain 100mg of THC in the amount advertised, contained anywhere from 50mg to 140mg of THC! So your "dose" of 10mg could be anywhere from 5mg to 14 mg. The other concern is the desire for some reason to sell very potent edibles. One candy bar tested by the Denver Post was advertised as containing 180mg of THC – and when tested it was found that it did indeed contain 180mg of THC. As the Post asked: "How exactly do you cut a candy bar into 18 pieces, and once you do, how do you eat just one piece and not end up eating more"?

Medical Marijuana

A follow-up study done this year – after several accidental deaths, a murder, and a suicide associated with edibles overdoses – reveals that the dispensaries are getting much better at managing the doses in the edibles, with few being higher than advertised. There is still a push to make edibles as single-dose servings.

Would you take a generic white pill that someone offered you if all they could tell you was that it would make you "high – maybe a little, maybe a lot"? That seems pretty foolish to me.

SAFE USE OF EDIBLES requires you to know what you are ingesting! You can't go to the dispensary and buy a couple of cookies, a "Rice-Krispie Treat", a brownie, and some "Jolly Ranchers" and know what you are going to get when you eat these various treats. I advise my patients to either make their own infused vegetable oil (if they grow their own marijuana) or to buy the infused oil from the dispensary. This oil can be used in any recipe requiring oil, such as a bag of brownie mix or cookie mix. Either brownies or cookies can be put in a plastic container and stored in the freezer. The key is that when you make a batch, *all of the cookies or brownies will have the same dose.* So make a batch, and start with a small serving half an hour before bed (or earlier in the evening if you need). Wait until the next day to assess how the dose worked for you. Again – all of the cookies or brownies will have the same dose.

A nice thing about edibles is that it is an inexpensive way of getting medical marijuana. Our local dispensary sells a small bottle of vegetable oil for $40. That is not bad for a batch of cookies that may have 20 to 40 doses.

Responsibility with edibles is vital! A few years ago in Maine a 12-year old took some of his mom's marijuana brownies to school and shared them with his buddies. Both he and his mom swear that he did not know that they were mom's marijuana brownies. I don't believe that for a minute – these brownies no longer have the hay texture of days gone by, but the infused oil or butter used to make them has a very strong "skunky" marijuana smell and taste. You would not bite in to one of these and continue eating it if you expected it to be a normal brownie!

In the case in Maine, all of the kids got stoned and were all kicked out of school. The young man who brought the brownies was taken into custody by the state and his mom was arrested and charged with endangering a child. The boy was placed in the foster system for three months! This put the family through hell. The state wanted to send a very strong message that this sort of behavior would absolutely not be tolerated. So – edibles should be very carefully kept out of reach of those who should not be eating them. I would hate to think of someone unknowingly eating a high-dose edible and then getting in their car for a four-hour drive!

And some people are just whacko about edibles. Patients all the time tell me that they use marijuana butter on bread and that they make all sorts of things using marijuana butter or oil. If I was using medical marijuana I don't really think the taste is all that pleasant to want everything I eat to taste that way.

I saw a patient not too long ago who was telling me how he had friends over the week before – apparently for an evening of relaxation or partying involving marijuana. "I made marijuana lasagna" he said. OK, I thought to myself....that is just totally wrong on four or five levels! First – I like lasagna, and it should taste like lasagna – tomato, cheese, some fresh basil, maybe a little fennel seed and some Italian Sausage – it should NOT taste like skunk! Second...if you are serving me this marijuana lasagna, how do I know what dose I am getting? Answer is I don't! I wouldn't like that at all. Third – what if the lasagna is tasty and I would like seconds....but I don't necessarily want to be twice as stoned! Fourth – if the goal is to get buzzed and go watch a movie or listen to music, the marijuana lasagna is going to take an hour before people are feeling it. Better to just pass a joint or bong or vape around. And fifth – the big one – unless he was having a great big sleep-over – his friends are still going to be stoned four or five hours later when they might expect to be driving home. If he had passed a joint around, by 11PM or midnight they would probably be safe to drive.

SO THINK, PEOPLE!

Tincture is the traditional way of consuming plant medicines by mouth. Traditionally tinctures are made by soaking the plant in alcohol for a few weeks to extract the desired compounds, and then this is run through a filter, and the tincture is given by the dropper or teaspoon.

> Recently in the Amazon I was visiting with a shaman. He had rows of used 2-liter soda bottles, each of which contained a special collection of leaves, roots, bark, flowers, etc. These bottles were then filled with alcohol and allowed to sit for a few weeks. When a patient presented with a problem, such as diarrhea, he knew which bottle contained the plants necessary for treating that, and he poured the patient a small glass. Pretty potent stuff. Perhaps if it didn't make you well you still might not care as much.

Tinctures made with alcohol have several advantages. First, strong alcohol often does a good job of extracting the compounds you want. Not all chemicals are soluble in water.

The other advantage of an alcohol-based tincture is that it will last indefinitely. The high alcohol content prevents the growth of mold or bacteria. It is still advisable to store it in a dark, cool place.

High up in the Andes Mountains, in Cusco, Peru, the cafes sell a lot of coca-leaf tea to the tourists, supposedly to help them acclimate to the 11,300 foot elevation – and that's at the *bottom* of the valley! What they don't bother to tell the tourists is that the active ingredient, a coca alkaloid, is **not** water-soluble! The local Quechua people wrap a coca leaf in some ash or ground limestone and hold it in their cheek. The alkalinity then converts the coca alkaloids into a water-soluble chemical that has mild stimulant activity. Likewise, THC and CBD are not very soluble in water, so a marijuana tea would not be very effective. However, this can be an advantage - some of the "skunky" flavor/smell chemicals are water soluble, so some people use water when they heat marijuana up with oil or butter to make an infusion. This helps the leaf material settle out and may reduce the off-taste. When chilled the butter hardens on top of the water.

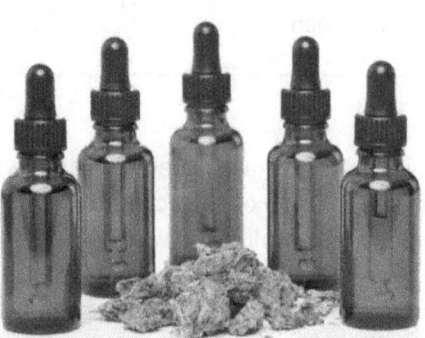

The dispensaries do not make and sell alcohol-based tinctures, however. They would probably need a federal liquor license to do so, and THAT ain't gonna happen! The dispensaries make tincture out of glycerin, a clear, syrupy, natural liquid. This can be fairly potent, but probably only has a shelf life of a few months unless refrigerated. A dropper-full can be placed under the tongue and held there (after a while you will have to swallow it).

Tincture has the advantage, like a big batch of home-made edibles, of being the same dose, so once you know what dose works for you, it is easily repeatable.

The problem with tincture is the taste: marijuana is a very smelly plant, often described as "skunky". Tincture tastes just like the plant smells. If you make your own, you can use a more flowery kush strain, but I hear very mixed reviews of the tincture from the dispensary. A few (very few...) patients tell me they love their tincture. One gentleman with back pain told me he looks forward to taking a dropper full of his tincture every night about half an hour before bed. "By bedtime I am out of pain and ready to sleep". He says he looks at it like his "dessert". But his reaction to tincture is not the average – most patients tell me they cannot stand the strong taste of tincture, and a few have told me they spit it out and immediately threw away the bottle of tincture they just spent $40 on. "Never again will I put that in my mouth!" they tell me.

However – many people tolerate homemade tincture a little better. If you make it yourself you can use alcohol, and you can do a lot to cover up the taste. Traditionally, 195-proof grain alcohol is used, but that is only available in a few states (as "Everclear" brand). You can get 151-proof Everclear or 151-proof rum in most states. 151-proof is 75.5% alcohol, which is strong enough to make tincture.

Dr. Blythe's Rum Tincture:

- Freeze 1 ounce leaf or bud in the freezer for 4 hours. Bud is more expensive but makes a much stronger tincture.
- Remove it from the freezer and crush well or pulverize with a blender or food processor.
- Put it in a 1-guart canning jar.
- Cover with 151-proof rum
- Let sit for two weeks, shaking once daily.
- Filter through a paper coffee filter.
- Store in an air-tight bottle.

Options: you can get cinnamon oil and add a few drops to the bottle to flavor the tincture. You can use this tincture mixed with juice, water, chocolate milk, or any liquid to help cover the taste. Some of my patients mix this tincture with a shot of spiced rum and have it on ice as a night-cap. Start with ¼ to ½ teaspoon of tincture and adjust if needed, making small changes daily until you find a good dose.

Medical Marijuana

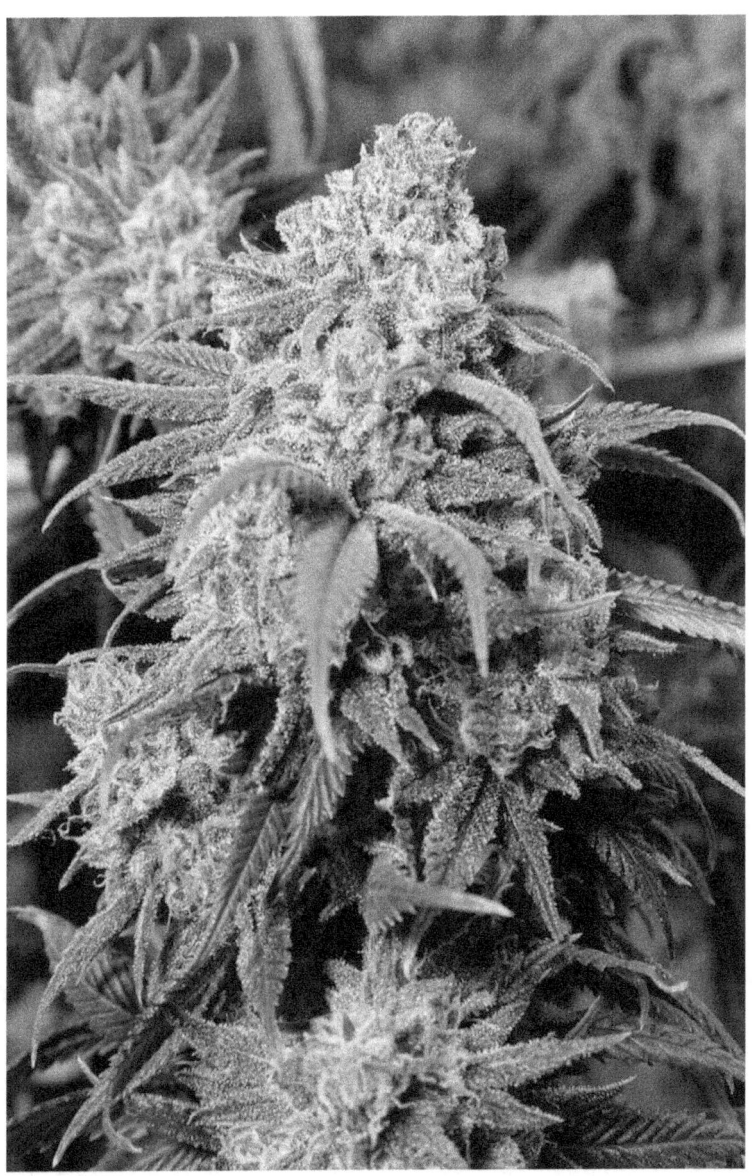

Chapter 6: Brief Pharmacology Overview

Marijuana contains a dozen or more biologically active "cannabinoid" compounds, but the two most important are tetrahydrocannabinol (THC) and cannabidiol (CBD). The reason these compounds work in our bodies is that we have naturally-occurring chemical hormones in our bodies that are similar to the cannabinoids. So when we introduce marijuana into our bodies, the THC and CBD act upon these receptors. CBD may also somewhat stimulate the serotonin receptors, thus helping reduce anxiety and depression. This could explain why states that have enacted medical marijuana laws have seen a decline in suicide rates. CBD has positive effects on cannabinoid receptors in the intestinal tract, and has been shown to lower the incidence of seizures. CBD also has been shown to have some anti-inflammatory effects. THC, on the other hand, seems to be more responsible for the "high" and some of the head effects. The interesting thing is that the cannabinoid receptors in the body have a greater affinity for CBD than for THC, so CBD, although generally in lesser quantity than THC in most strains, actually blocks some of the effect of THC. So – the impact of any given marijuana strain or plant will be not just a function of how much THC and CBD, but in the ratio, or relative amount, of each.

Chapter 7: Strainology

When someone gets illegal marijuana, what they get is whatever they *can* get. It is whatever their "guy" has to offer. With legal marijuana, a patient has the option and new-found freedom to try different strains to see what strain works best for their condition. That is one of the really neat things about legalizing medical marijuana.

There are two main species of the genus *Cannabis: Cannabis sativa* and *Cannabis indica*. The *C. sativa* was first identified in western botanical literature in 1753 by Linnaeus, although it had been cultivated for thousands of years.

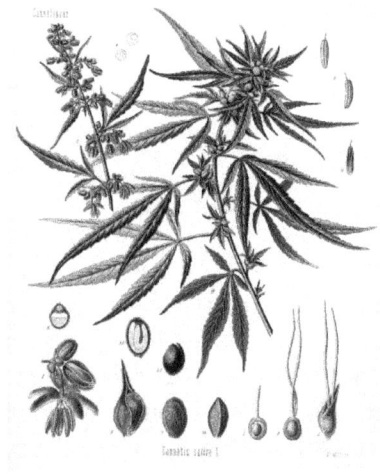

Wood block print of Cannabis sativa from the 1800's.

This is a most versatile plant: the seeds can be crushed for oil and used for feed, and the stems can be used to make hemp, for centuries the main constituent of ropes and fabric. Medicinal use is spotty in recorded literature. The *C. indica* species, originally from the Hindu Kush region of India, was identified in 1785.

In the 1960's the U.S. government undertook a massive program to eradicate wild-growing Cannabis in the Midwestern United States. Some estimates are that this caused up to a 50% decline in the songbird population of the U.S., since hempseed was a major winter food source for these birds.

There are important differences between indica and sativa:

Pharmacology: Indica tends to have relatively more CBD than sativa. This means that indica strains are generally better than sativa strains for treatment of pain and inflammation, including inflammatory bowel disease. Sativa strains are lower in CBD, and thus are probably better for treating anxiety, PTSD, and OCD. Both strains appear to help nausea, vomiting, and appetite. Strains of indica such as R4 which are very high in CBD are often used to treat seizure disorders in children because there is not enough THC to cause any sort of "high". Some states have even legalized medical marijuana only if there is a very high CBD-to-THC ratio.

So – you can narrow down your choice to sativa or indica, but there are hundreds of strains of each, and even hybrids combining the properties of sativa and indica! How do you find the best strain for your condition? The simplest way will be working with your dispensary – because you are of course limited to the strains they have. I have found the employees of the dispensaries to be very knowledgeable about the strains they offer. If you want to grow your own or have a caregiver grow for you, you can seek seeds or cuttings of various strains to grow.

There are several good websites which review the various strains:

> www.leafly.com
> www.medicalmarijuanastrains.com
> http://www.thecannabist.co/

The last website is a resource in Colorado which also has lots of articles of general interest, recipes, etc.

Growth characteristics: of *sativa* and indica are different. *Indicas* tend to be shorter and more dense, and so are better-suited for growing indoors. *Indicas* are also better-suited for cooler, temperate climates. *Sativas* do well indoors, but may grow six or eight feet high, thus being a challenge to grow in your living room.

Cannabis requires long periods of daylight – more than 12-13 hours daily – during its growth phase. When the daylight hours start to grow shorter it will enter the flowering phase, which may take months.

Chapter 8: Getting Your Medical Marijuana in Maine

Some states allow the growing of marijuana by legal patients, others do not. The law in Maine requires anyone growing marijuana outdoors to do so behind a six-foot privacy fence which has a gate locked with a padlock and which has motion-activated security lighting. Growing indoors does not pose such a security risk.

Also, in Maine, those who grow may grow up to six mature plants at a time. They may have any number of seedlings, but as the seedlings get to the stage of budding, there needs to be just six plants. Legal Maine medical marijuana patients may possess up to 2.5 ounces of *processed* marijuana – but if you grow, you are most likely going to have more than that when you harvest your plants. That is OK – Maine law *allows you to have up to eight pounds* of harvested marijuana, as long as it is not processed for use – it must still be on the stem. This is a generous concession to those who can only grow one outdoor crop per year.

Six plants is the magic number. Either you can grow six plants, or you can designate someone else to grow them for you. Or you can share the pleasure and/or responsibility.

Maine allows others (who might have a greenhouse and/or a greener thumb than you) to grow marijuana for you. These folks are called "caregivers" by the Maine Medical Marijuana Program. A caregiver must be licensed by the state, must pay a tax/fee for each patient they grow for, and can grow up to six plants for up to five patients who designate them to do so. Being a caregiver has become quite a cottage industry in the state – many folks make a little extra money on the side through their horticultural endeavors. Some of them even have many years of experience growing marijuana! Now they can turn that experience into a legal source of fun and profit! Some caregivers make edibles for their customers, and some deliver to their customers who are disabled.

When you become certified in Maine, the new system results in your getting **two cards**. One is your "Certification" which makes it legal for you to buy, grow, and possess medical marijuana. The other card is your "Designation" card. If you grow your own marijuana, you can just hold on to this card. If someone else grows marijuana for you, you must provide them with this designation card – whether that is the dispensary or your caregiver. *You only get one designation card* – you cannot have more than one caregiver and you cannot use both a dispensary AND a caregiver. If you wish to change, the caregiver or dispensary you are using must return the card to you.

Splitting the difference: you can grow some plants AND have someone else grow for you. Since caregivers are limited to five customers/patients, they may not be very interested in taking you on if you do not have a significant need for their product. But many people grow some plants and also use a dispensary where they can buy edibles, try different strains, buy other supplies (such as the O-pen Vape), etc. When you first sign up with a dispensary or caregiver you are required to complete a designation form. It requires you to specifically state how many plants you will be growing and how many plants you designate the caregiver or dispensary to grow on your behalf. Of course, if you only designate one or two plants to the dispensary they are not going to be willing to sell you large volumes of marijuana. One dispensary posts a sign saying that if you only designate them one or two plants the most you can purchase is one-half ounce every two weeks.

Medical Marijuana

Finding a Certifying Professional: In Maine either a physician (an M.D. or a D.O.) or a nurse practitioner can provide your certification. A physician's assistant is not permitted to do this. The new system guarantees that the person doing your certificate is authorized to do so. Under the old system anyone who had some tamper-proof paper could print up and sign a certification for you. And some who did were not authorized to do so! One PA from out-of-state set up shop in Bangor and "sold" a lot of certificates. When the state started sniffing around, he left town. All of the dispensaries received letters advising them not toaccept any certificates signed by him (he was at least smart enough to sign the certificates with the name of the doctor "he was working with"). Likewise was a gynecologist who apparently had gotten into trouble with the licensing board over his prescribing practices and who as part of his punishment had signed a consent decree agreeing to limit his practice to outpatient gynecology. He then started doing MMJ certifications. The licensing board was none too happy about that, and the Department of Health advised dispensaries not to accept his certificates. Sadly, the ones punished were those who had paid him $300 to get a certificate.

Unfortunately, given the federal standing of medical marijuana, and the fact that almost all medical institutions in Maine rely heavily on federal support, most physicians and nurse practitioners in the state have been advised (or told...) not to issue medical marijuana certifications. Only about 3% of the physicians in fact will certify their patients. I finally decided to start providing this service to patients other than my own on a consulting basis because I was seeing patients who were driving eight hours round trip and paying $300 to get certified. I thought that was a bit excessive.

What is required to get certified: Physicians and nurse practitioners who certify patients who are not their regular patients have different requirements for providing the certification. Based on the qualifying condition, the requirement may be easily met or may be a challenge. I have outlined **my** requirements for certifying a patient.

Pain: This can be a challenge. The state requires an MMJ patient to have "chronic intractable pain" which is "not responding to customary treatment". Any time we treat pain we cannot tell just how much pain someone actually is having. While I do not assume that this requirement necessarily means that a patient is using oxycodone or has had surgery, I do require medical records that document that the patient has sought evaluation and/or relief for their painful condition. I have had people request MMJ for "ear pain" for which they had never seen a doctor. One patient presented records which consisted of an x-ray showing a broken ankle twenty years previously. Perhaps it still hurts when it rains, but I did not think that he qualified. An MRI showing "moderate to severe" degenerative disc disease would be enough to convince me that someone had pain, although recently someone who advised me that his MRI showed "severe" problems with his back brought me a report which documented "mild degenerative disc disease" – which is something that almost anyone over 50 has in their spine. It does *not* indicate pain. I will accept office records showing multiple visits for chiropractic treatment or physical therapy as an indicator of chronic pain. I also will accept a referral form from their treating provider documenting that they are under care for chronic pain. Especially any patient receiving opioid medications should clear the use of MMJ with their provider so that there will not be problems when a urine drug screen shows positive results for THC.

PTSD: I am not a psychologist or psychiatrist. You can tell me that you have PTSD all you want, but I do not know that. I will be happy to certify someone with a referral from their mental health provider documenting that they are under their care for PTSD. The VA physicians are not only unwilling to certify patients for MMJ but are unwilling to sign any referral forms for my practice, but I will accept any documentation of a PTSD diagnosis from the VA. This includes a veteran's discharge paperwork saying that they have some degree of disability from PTSD. Otherwise it is pretty easy for vets to go online and get copies of their medical records.

Crohn's Disease: I like to get some office notes or a referral documenting that someone is under treatment for inflammatory bowel disease. I had an urgent consultation with a patient who had to go out of town and who did not have his records. His colostomy bag and an abdomen covered with surgical scars were fairly convincing that he had suffered from Crohn's for a number of years.

Hepatitis C: While a referral from a provider is useful, some providers are not well-schooled on Hepatitis C. I have had referrals for patients *who did not actually have Hepatitis C.* So, I advised them of the "good news, bad news" that they did not qualify for MMJ, but that they did NOT have Hepatitis C. This is because there are two blood tests needed to diagnose Hepatitis C. The Hepatitis C *antibody test* will indicate whether or not you have ever been exposed to the virus. Most people who are exposed and who develop antibodies go on to develop chronic Hepatitis C infection. They are contagious (through blood-sharing only) and need to be further evaluated, monitored, and at some point treated (there is a new but very, very expensive treatment). But some people who are exposed are able to fight off the virus and never develop chronic Hepatitis C. This is determined by a *viral load* test. This is a very sensitive test to look for genetic material from the Hepatitis C virus in the bloodstream. If you have none, then you do not have the disease. If it is positive, then you do in fact have Hepatitis C. *I require a copy of both test results to verify Hepatitis C.* By the way, anyone who has ever shared needles or who has had a transfusion before 1991 who has not been screened should consider screening. Getting a tattoo in an unlicensed setting such as prison or an underdeveloped country would count as "sharing needles".

Anxiety, insomnia, and/or Depression: I often receive referrals for patients with these diagnoses. They are *not* qualifying conditions under the Maine Medical Marijuana Program, however.

Other conditions: cancer, chemotherapy, MS, and other degenerative conditions or treatments causing nausea, loss of appetite, or muscle spasm all require medical records documenting the condition or a referral form completed by the patient's provider.

But Isn't Marijuana a "Gateway Drug"?

In this year before elections, there are a few seeking elected office that promise to reverse and undo a lot of the forward movement that has happened with medical marijuana. Their argument is that it is a "gateway drug" – that using marijuana will lead to using harder drugs. It was this concern that helped derail Florida's Medical Marijuana referendum in 2014.

If marijuana is a gateway drug then why isn't beer a gateway drug? Why isn't Coca-Cola a gateway drug – surely those who want some natural mild stimulant effect would next start using cocaine!

If marijuana leads to the use of harder drugs, it is only because of it being illegal. The person from whom you are forced to buy your marijuana may indeed have other things they would like to sell to you. The fact that you are engaging in an illegal activity might in the minds of some people make it that much easier to make the step to another illegal substance. If you can get life in prison in Texas for possession of some hash brownies, what difference does it really make if you have a few baggies of heroin in your pocket? Are they going to add no a few more years?

Clearly some people have addictive personalities. Those people probably have more trouble with the progression from beer to alcoholism than they have with marijuana.

One can argue that there will be less use of hard drugs if those who simply want to get a buzz from marijuana – and certainly those who want to treat their pain, PTSD, or other illness – are not forced to conduct business with drug dealers.

There is no rational argument against the legalization of medical marijuana. As a physician I can prescribe you oxycodone. I can prescribe you amphetamine. I can even prescribe you pure, synthetic THC. But in half the states I cannot advise you to use a safe, natural plant medicine that has been used for millennia!

It is time for that to change!

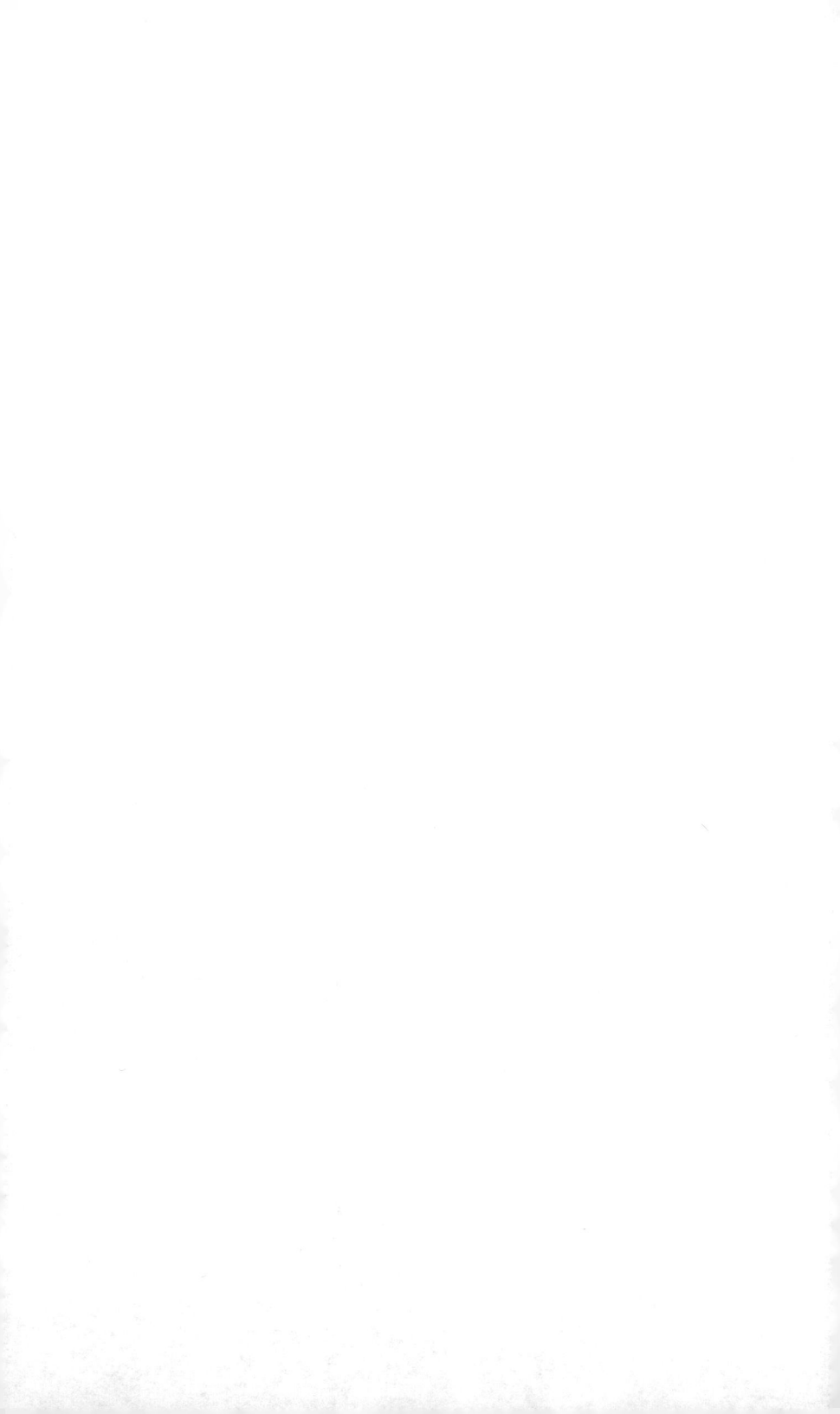